RHEUMATOID ARTHRITIS DIET COOKBOOK FOR SENIORS

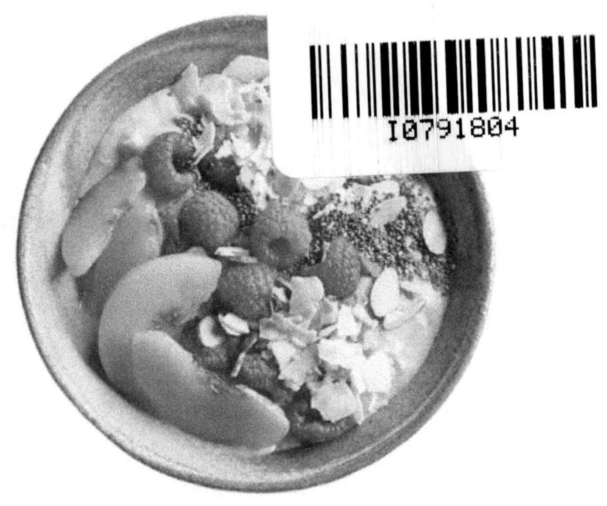

Delicious Anti Inflammatory Recipes for Managing Rheumatoid Arthritis in Older Adults

Linda Carlucci

Copyright © 2024 by Linda Carlucci

DISCLAIMER

This cookbook is intended to provide general information and recipes.

The recipes provided in this cookbook are not intended to replace or be a substitute for medical advice from a physician.

The reader should consult a healthcare professional for any specific medical advice, diagnosis or treatment.

Any specific dietary advice provided in this cookbook is not intended to replace or be a substitute for medical advice from a physician.

The author is not responsible or liable for any adverse effects experienced by readers of this cookbook as a result of following the recipes or dietary advice provided.

The author makes no representations or warranties of any kind (express or implied) as to the accuracy, completeness, reliability or suitability of the recipes provided in this cookbook.

The author disclaims any and all liability for any damages arising out of the use or misuse of the recipes provided in this cookbook. The reader must also take care to ensure that the recipes provided in this cookbook are prepared and cooked safely.

The recipes provided in this cookbook are for informational purposes only and should not be used as a substitute for professional medical advice, diagnosis or treatment.

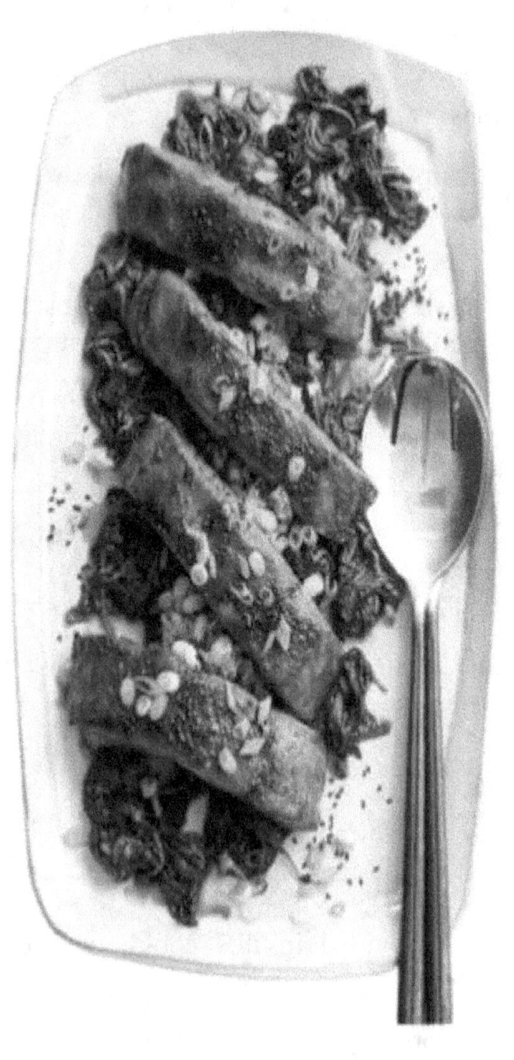

TABLE OF CONTENTS

INTRODUCTION

Rheumatoid arthritis (RA) is a persistent inflammatory condition that mainly impacts the joints. While there's no specific diet to cure RA, certain foods can help manage symptoms and improve overall health.

A well-balanced diet rich in nutrients can support the immune system, reduce inflammation, and maintain a healthy weight, all of which are crucial for managing RA.

One key aspect of an RA diet is incorporating anti-inflammatory foods.

These include fatty fish like salmon, mackerel, and sardines, which are high in omega-3 fatty acids.

Omega-3s have been shown to reduce inflammation and may help relieve RA symptoms.

Other anti-inflammatory foods include fruits, vegetables, whole grains, nuts, and seeds.

On the flip side, it's important to limit foods that can increase inflammation. These consist of processed foods, refined sugars, and saturated fats. Reducing the intake of these foods can help manage RA symptoms and improve overall health.

Some people with RA may also benefit from following a Mediterranean-style diet, which emphasizes fruits, vegetables, whole grains, legumes, nuts, and olive oil.

This diet is rich in antioxidants and anti-inflammatory compounds, which can help reduce inflammation and improve symptoms.

In addition to diet, staying hydrated is important for people with RA.

Drinking plenty of water can help maintain joint function and reduce inflammation.

While diet can play a role in managing RA, it's important to work with a healthcare provider or a registered dietitian to develop a personalized plan.

They can help you identify foods that may trigger inflammation or aggravate symptoms and create a diet that meets your nutritional needs while managing RA.

CHAPTER 1

COMMON CAUSES OF RHEUMATOID ARTHRITIS IN SENIORS

1. **Genetics:** There is a genetic component to RA, and seniors with a family history of the disease are at a higher risk of developing it.

2. **Age:** Aging is a risk factor for RA. As people age, the immune system may weaken, making them more susceptible to autoimmune diseases like RA.

3. **Environmental Factors:** Exposure to certain environmental factors, such as smoking, pollution, or infections, may increase the risk of developing RA, especially in seniors.

4. **Hormones:** Changes in hormone levels, particularly in women after menopause, may contribute to the development of RA.

5. **Lifestyle Factors:** Factors such as obesity, sedentary lifestyle, and poor diet may increase the risk of developing RA in seniors.

6. **Other Medical Conditions:** Seniors with certain medical conditions, such as gum disease, may have an increased risk of developing RA.

RISK FACTORS OF RHEUMATOID ARTHRITIS IN SENIORS

1. **Age:** The risk of developing RA increases with age, especially in seniors over 60 years old.
2. **Gender:** Women are more likely to develop RA than men, and this difference is more pronounced in older age groups.
3. **Genetics:** A family history of RA or other autoimmune diseases increases the risk of developing RA.
4. **Smoking:** Smoking is a significant risk factor for RA, especially in seniors.
5. **Obesity:** Excess weight puts added stress on the joints, increasing the risk of developing RA.
6. **Environmental Factors:** Exposure to certain environmental factors, such as pollution or infections, may increase the risk of developing RA.

7. **Hormones:** Changes in hormone levels, particularly in women after menopause, may contribute to the development of RA.

8. **Lifestyle Factors:** Factors such as sedentary lifestyle, poor diet, and high levels of stress may increase the risk of developing RA in seniors.

9. **Other Medical Conditions:** Seniors with certain medical conditions, such as gum disease, may have an increased risk of developing RA.

FOODS TO AVOID FOR SENIORS WITH RHEUMATOID ARTHRITIS

1. **Processed Foods:** These often contain high levels of unhealthy fats, sugars, and additives that can contribute to inflammation.

2. **Saturated Fats:** Found in red meat, full-fat dairy products, and some processed foods, saturated fats can increase inflammation.

3. **Trans Fats:** Found in fried foods, baked goods, and margarine, trans fats can also increase inflammation and worsen RA symptoms.

4. **Sugar and High-Glycemic Foods:** These can cause spikes in blood sugar levels, which may contribute to inflammation.

5. **Refined Carbohydrates:** White bread, white rice, and pasta can also lead to increased inflammation.

6. **Alcohol:** Excessive alcohol consumption can contribute to inflammation and may interact with medications used to treat RA.

7. **Nightshade Vegetables:** Some people with RA find that vegetables like tomatoes, peppers, eggplants, and potatoes worsen their symptoms, although more research is needed in this area.

LIST OF ANTI-INFLAMMATORY HERBS AND SPICES

1. **Turmeric:** Contains curcumin, which has strong anti-inflammatory properties. It's been used in traditional medicine for centuries to treat inflammatory conditions.

2. **Ginger:** Contains gingerol, which has anti-inflammatory effects. It's commonly used to reduce inflammation and relieve pain.

3. **Cinnamon:** Contains antioxidants and has anti-inflammatory properties. It may help reduce inflammation and lower the risk of chronic diseases.

4. **Cloves:** Contain eugenol, a compound with anti-inflammatory properties. Cloves have been used in traditional medicine to treat inflammatory conditions.

5. **Garlic:** Contains sulfur compounds with anti-inflammatory effects. It may help reduce inflammation and lower the risk of chronic diseases.

6. **Cayenne Pepper:** Contains capsaicin, which has anti-inflammatory properties. It's often used topically to relieve pain and inflammation.

7. **Rosemary:** Contains carnosol and rosmarinic acid, which have anti-inflammatory effects. Rosemary extract has been shown to reduce inflammation in several studies.

8. **Thyme:** Contains thymol, which has anti-inflammatory properties. It's often used in cooking and traditional medicine to reduce inflammation.

9. **Oregano:** Contains carvacrol, a compound with anti-inflammatory effects.

10. **Sage:** Contains rosmarinic acid, which has anti-inflammatory properties. Sage extract has been shown to reduce inflammation in several studies.

BENEFITS OF FOLLOWING AN ANTI-INFLAMMATORY DIET FOR MANAGING RHEUMATOID ARTHRITI

1. **Reduced Inflammation:** An anti-inflammatory diet can help reduce inflammation in the body, which is a key factor in RA. Foods like fatty fish, leafy greens, and berries contain anti-inflammatory compounds that can help alleviate RA symptoms.

2. **Improved Joint Health:** By reducing inflammation, an anti-inflammatory diet can help improve joint health and reduce pain, swelling, and stiffness associated with RA.

3. **Weight Management:** Many anti-inflammatory foods are also low in calories and can help with weight management. Maintaining a healthy weight is important for managing RA, as excess weight can put added stress on the joints.

4. **Heart Health:** Some anti-inflammatory foods, such as fatty fish and nuts, are also good for heart health. People with RA have an increased risk of heart disease, so maintaining heart health is important.

5. **Nutrient-Rich Foods:** An anti-inflammatory diet emphasizes nutrient-rich foods like fruits, vegetables, whole grains, and lean proteins, which can help support overall health and boost the immune system.

6. **Improved Gut Health:** Some studies suggest that an anti-inflammatory diet can improve gut health, which may be beneficial for people with RA, as gut health is linked to inflammation and immune function.

7. **Better Overall Health:** By promoting a balanced diet rich in nutrients, an anti-inflammatory diet can help improve overall health and well-being, which is important for managing a chronic condition like RA.

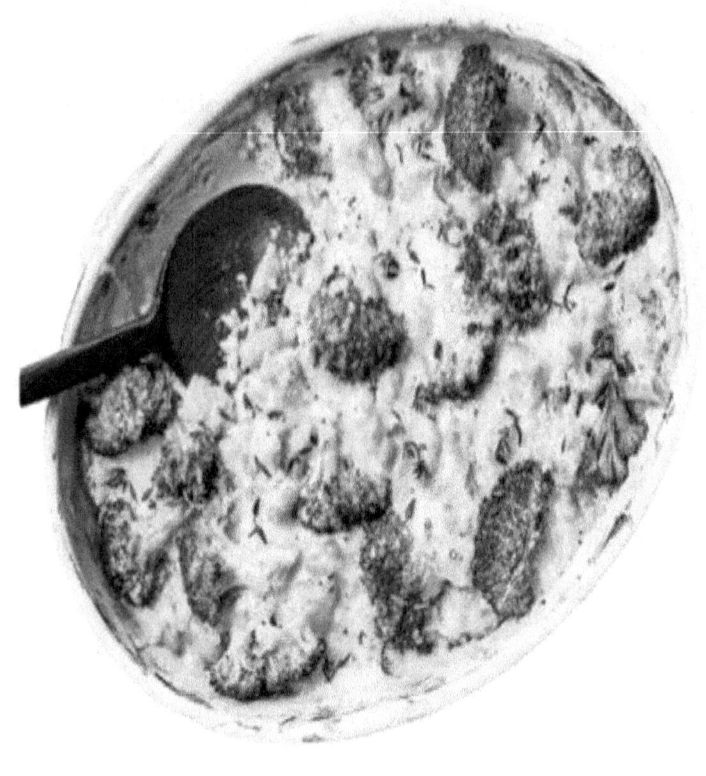

14-DAY MEAL PLAN

DAY 1

Breakfast: Greek Yogurt with Fruit

Lunch: Salmon Rice Bowl

Dinner: Chicken & Spinach Skillet Pasta with Lemon & Parmesan

DAY 2

Breakfast: Salmon Omelet

Lunch: Vegetarian Protein Bowl

Dinner: Spinach & Mushroom Quiche

DAY 3

Breakfast: Almond Butter with Vegetable Sticks

Lunch: Green Goddess Sandwich

Dinner: Crispy Rice Bowls with Fried Eggs

DAY 4

Breakfast: Spinach, Mushroom & Egg Casserole

Lunch: Vegan Burrito Bowls with Cauliflower Rice

Dinner: Gochujang-Glazed Salmon with Garlic Spinach

DAY 5

Breakfast: Lemon-Blueberry Yogurt Toast

Lunch: Vegan Burrito Bowls with Cauliflower Rice

Dinner: Broccoli & Quinoa Casserole

DAY 6

Breakfast: Frittata with Asparagus, Leek & Ricotta

Lunch: Pesto Chicken Quinoa Bowls

Dinner: Salmon with Lemon-Herb Orzo & Broccoli

DAY 7

Breakfast: Mixed-Berry Breakfast Smoothie

Lunch: Farro Salad with Arugula, Artichokes & Pistachios

Dinner: Easy Salmon Cakes with Arugula Salad

DAY 8

Breakfast: Muffin-Tin Spinach & Mushroom Mini Quiche

Lunch: Salmon-Stuffed Avocados

Dinner: Salmon & Asparagus with Lemon-Garlic Butter Sauce

DAY 9

Breakfast: Spinach & Egg Scramble with Raspberries

Lunch: Winter Kale & Quinoa Salad with Avocado

Dinner: Skillet Lemon Chicken with Spinach

DAY 10

Breakfast: Muffin-Tin Omelets with Black Beans and Jack Cheese

Lunch: Green Goddess Salad with Chickpeas

Dinner: Broccoli and Turkey Sausage Skillet Pizza

DAY 11

Breakfast: Greek Yogurt with Fruit

Lunch: Salmon Rice Bowl

Dinner: Chicken & Spinach Skillet Pasta with Lemon & Parmesan

DAY 12

Breakfast: Salmon Omelet

Lunch: Vegetarian Protein Bowl

Dinner: Spinach & Mushroom Quiche

DAY 13

Breakfast: Almond Butter with Vegetable Sticks

Lunch: Green Goddess Sandwich

Dinner: Crispy Rice Bowls with Fried Eggs

DAY 14

Breakfast: Spinach, Mushroom & Egg Casserole

Lunch: Vegan Burrito Bowls with Cauliflower Rice

Dinner: Gochujang-Glazed Salmon with Garlic Spinach

CHAPTER 3

NUTRITIOUS RECIPES FOR A RHEUMATOID ARTHRITIS DIET

BREAKFAST

Greek Yogurt with Fruit

Preparation Time: 5 minutes

Serves: 1

Calories: 230 **Carbs:** 30g **Protein:** 20g **Fat:** 2g **Fiber:** 3g **Sodium:** 60mg

Ingredients:

1 cup Greek yogurt

1/2 cup mixed berries (such as strawberries, blueberries, and raspberries)

1 tablespoon honey

1/4 teaspoon cinnamon

Method of Preparation:

1. In a bowl, mix the Greek yogurt with honey and cinnamon.
2. Top with mixed berries.
3. Serve and enjoy!

Salmon Omelet

Preparation Time: 10 minutes

Serves: 1

Calories: 300 **Carbs:** 5g **Protein:** 25g **Fat:** 20g **Fiber:** 2g **Sodium:** 100mg

Ingredients:

2 eggs

1/4 cup cooked salmon, flaked

1/4 cup spinach, chopped

1/4 teaspoon garlic powder

1/4 teaspoon paprika

Method of Preparation:

1. In a bowl, whisk the eggs with garlic powder, and paprika.
2. Heat a non-stick skillet over medium heat and pour in the egg mixture.
3. Cook for 2-3 minutes, then add the flaked salmon, and spinach.
4. Fold the omelet in half and cook for another 2-3 minutes, or until the eggs are fully cooked.
5. Serve hot.

Almond Butter With Vegetable Sticks

Preparation Time: 5 minutes

Serves: 1

Calories: 250 **Carbs:** 20g **Protein:** 7g **Fat:** 17g **Fiber:** 8g **Sodium:** 50mg

Ingredients:

2 tablespoons almond butter

1 medium carrot, cut into sticks

1 medium cucumber, cut into sticks

Method of Preparation:

1. Place almond butter in a small bowl for dipping.
2. Serve with carrot sticks, and cucumber sticks.
3. Enjoy as a healthy snack.

Spinach, Mushroom & Egg Casserole

Preparation Time: 50 minutes

Serves: 6

Calories: 180 **Carbs:** 6g **Protein:** 14g **Fat:** 11g **Fiber:** 1g **Sodium:** 150mg

Ingredients:

8 eggs

1/2 cup milk

1 cup spinach, chopped

1 cup mushrooms, sliced

1/2 cup onion, diced

1/2 cup shredded mozzarella cheese

1/2 teaspoon garlic powder

1/2 teaspoon paprika

Cooking spray

Method of Preparation:

1. Preheat oven to 350°F (175°C) and grease a baking dish with cooking spray.
2. In a large bowl, whisk together eggs, milk, garlic powder, and paprika.
3. Stir in spinach, mushrooms, onion, and mozzarella cheese.
4. Pour mixture into the prepared baking dish and bake for 25-30 minutes, or until eggs are set.
5. Allow to cool slightly before serving.

Lemon-Blueberry Yogurt Toast

Preparation Time: 5 minutes

Serves: 1

Calories: 280 **Carbs:** 50g **Protein:** 14g **Fat:** 3g **Fiber:** 6g
Sodium: 120mg

Ingredients:

2 slices whole grain bread

1/2 cup Greek yogurt

1/2 cup blueberries

1 tablespoon honey

1/2 teaspoon lemon zest

Method of Preparation:

1. Toast the bread slices until golden brown.
2. Spread Greek yogurt evenly over the toast.
3. Top with blueberries, drizzle with honey, and sprinkle with lemon zest.
4. Serve immediately.

Frittata with Asparagus, Leek & Ricotta

Preparation Time: 45 minutes

Serves: 4

Calories: 220 **Carbs:** 5g **Protein:** 16g **Fat:** 15g **Fiber:** 2g **Sodium:** 130mg

Ingredients:

6 eggs

1/2 cup ricotta cheese

1/2 cup asparagus, chopped

1/2 cup leek, sliced

1/4 cup Parmesan cheese, grated

1/2 teaspoon dried thyme

Cooking spray

Method of Preparation:

1. Preheat oven to 350°F (175°C).
2. In a large bowl, whisk together eggs, ricotta cheese, and dried thyme.
3. Heat a non-stick skillet over medium heat and coat with cooking spray.
4. Add asparagus and leek to the skillet and sauté until tender, about 5 minutes.
5. Pour egg mixture over the vegetables and cook for 2-3 minutes, or until the edges start to set.
6. Sprinkle Parmesan cheese over the top.

7. Transfer skillet to the preheated oven and bake for 15-20 minutes, or until eggs are fully set.

8. Allow to cool slightly before slicing and serving.

Mixed-Berry Breakfast Smoothie

Preparation Time: 5 minutes

Serves: 1

Calories: 250 **Carbs:** 35g **Protein:** 14g **Fat:** 6g **Fiber:** 8g **Sodium:** 90mg

Ingredients:

1/2 cup mixed berries (such as strawberries, blueberries, and raspberries)

1/2 banana

1/2 cup Greek yogurt

1/2 cup almond milk

1 tablespoon chia seeds

1 tablespoon honey (optional)

Method of Preparation:

1. Place all ingredients in a blender and blend until smooth.
2. Serve immediately.

Muffin-Tin Spinach & Mushroom Mini Quiches

Preparation Time: 35 minutes

Serves: 6

Calories: 120 **Carbs:** 3g **Protein:** 9g **Fat:** 8g **Fiber:** 1g **Sodium:** 80mg

Ingredients:

6 eggs

1/2 cup milk

1 cup spinach, chopped

1/2 cup mushrooms, sliced

1/4 cup onion, diced

1/2 cup shredded cheddar cheese

1/2 teaspoon garlic powder

Cooking spray

Method of Preparation:

1. Preheat oven to 350°F (175°C) and grease a muffin tin with cooking spray.
2. In a large bowl, whisk together eggs, milk, and garlic powder.
3. Stir in spinach, mushrooms, onion, and cheddar cheese.
4. Pour mixture into the prepared muffin tin and bake for 20-25 minutes, or until eggs are set.
5. Allow to cool slightly before serving.

Spinach & Egg Scramble with Raspberries

Preparation Time: 10 minutes

Serves: 1

Calories: 220 **Carbs:** 10g **Protein:** 12g **Fat:** 15g **Fiber:** 5g
Sodium: 110mg

Ingredients:

2 eggs

1 cup spinach

1/4 cup raspberries

1 tablespoon olive oil

1/2 teaspoon garlic powder

Method of Preparation:

1. Heat olive oil in a skillet over medium heat.
2. Add spinach and cook until wilted, about 2 minutes.
3. Whisk eggs with garlic powder and then pour into the skillet with the spinach.
4. Scramble eggs until cooked through, about 3-4 minutes.
5. Serve with raspberries on the side.

Muffin-Tin Omelets with Black Beans and Jack Cheese

Preparation Time: 35 minutes

Serves: 6

Calories: 150 **Carbs:** 6g **Protein:** 11g **Fat:** 9g **Fiber:** 2g **Sodium:** 100mg

Ingredients:

6 eggs

1/2 cup black beans, drained and rinsed

1/2 cup shredded Monterey Jack cheese

1/4 cup onion, diced

1/2 teaspoon garlic powder

Cooking spray

Method of Preparation:

1. Preheat oven to 350°F (175°C) and grease a muffin tin with cooking spray.
2. In a large bowl, whisk together eggs, and garlic powder.
3. Stir in black beans, cheese, and onion.
4. Pour mixture into the prepared muffin tin and bake for 20-25 minutes, or until eggs are set.
5. Allow to cool slightly before serving.

LUNCH

Salmon Rice Bowl

Preparation Time: 15 minutes

Serves: 1

Calories: 400 **Carbs:** 30g **Protein:** 30g **Fat:** 18g **Fiber:** 8g
Sodium: 60mg

Ingredients:

1/2 cup brown rice, cooked

4 oz salmon fillet

1/2 cup broccoli, steamed

1/2 cup carrots, shredded

1/4 avocado, sliced

1 tablespoon soy sauce

1 teaspoon sesame oil

1/2 teaspoon ginger, minced

1/2 teaspoon garlic, minced

Method of Preparation:

1. Season salmon fillet with ginger, and garlic.
2. In a skillet over medium heat, cook salmon for 3-4 minutes on each side, or until cooked through.
3. In a bowl, combine cooked rice, steamed broccoli, shredded carrots, and sliced avocado.
4. In a small bowl, mix soy sauce and sesame oil, then drizzle over the rice bowl.
5. Top with cooked salmon and serve.

Vegetarian Protein Bowl

Preparation Time: 15 minutes

Serves: 1

Calories: 400 **Carbs:** 45g **Protein:** 20g **Fat:** 16g **Fiber:** 12g **Sodium:** 90mg

Ingredients:

1/2 cup quinoa, cooked

1/2 cup chickpeas, drained and rinsed

1/2 cup edamame, shelled and cooked

1/4 cup cucumber, diced

1/4 cup feta cheese, crumbled

1 tablespoon olive oil

1 tablespoon lemon juice

1/2 teaspoon dried oregano

Method of Preparation:

1. In a bowl, combine cooked quinoa, chickpeas, edamame, cucumber, and feta cheese.
2. In a small bowl, whisk together olive oil, lemon juice, and oregano.
3. Drizzle dressing over the quinoa mixture and toss to combine.
4. Serve and enjoy!

Green Goddess Sandwich

Preparation Time: 10 minutes

Serves: 1

Calories: 350 **Carbs:** 45g **Protein:** 12g **Fat:** 15g **Fiber:** 12g
Sodium: 50mg

Ingredients:

2 slices whole grain bread

1/4 cup hummus

1/4 avocado, mashed

1/4 cup cucumber, sliced

1/4 cup spinach leaves

1/4 cup alfalfa sprouts

1 tablespoon lemon juice

1/2 teaspoon garlic powder

Method of Preparation:

1. Toast the bread slices until golden brown.
2. Spread hummus on one slice of bread and mashed avocado on the other slice.
3. Layer cucumber, spinach leaves, and alfalfa sprouts on one slice of bread.
4. Drizzle lemon juice over the vegetables and sprinkle with garlic powder.
5. Top with the other slice of bread and press gently to seal.

6. Slice in half and serve.

Vegan Burrito Bowls with Cauliflower Rice

Preparation Time: 15 minutes

Serves: 1

Calories: 300 **Carbs:** 45g **Protein:** 12g **Fat:** 10g **Fiber:** 12g
Sodium: 80mg

Ingredients:

1 cup cauliflower rice, cooked

1/2 cup black beans, drained and rinsed

1/2 cup corn kernels

1/4 cup red onion, diced

1/4 cup cilantro, chopped

1/2 avocado, sliced

1/2 lime, juiced

1/2 teaspoon cumin

1/2 teaspoon chili powder

A pinch of salt

Method of Preparation:

1. In a bowl, combine cauliflower rice, black beans, corn, red onion, cilantro, cumin, chili powder, salt, and lime juice.
2. Mix well to combine.
3. Top with avocado slices and serve.

Pesto Chicken Quinoa Bowls

Preparation Time: 35 minutes

Serves: 1

Calories: 400 **Carbs:** 35g **Protein:** 35g **Fat:** 15g **Fiber:** 5g **Sodium:** 90mg

Ingredients:

4 oz chicken breast

1/2 cup quinoa, cooked

1/4 cup cucumber, diced

1/4 cup red onion, diced

2 tablespoons pesto sauce

1 tablespoon lemon juice

1/2 teaspoon garlic powder

A pinch of salt

Method of Preparation:

1. Season chicken breast with garlic powder, and salt.
2. In a skillet over medium heat, cook chicken for 5-7 minutes on each side, or until cooked through.
3. In a bowl, combine cooked quinoa, cucumber, red onion, pesto sauce, and lemon juice.
4. Mix well to combine.
5. Slice chicken breast and serve over quinoa mixture.

Farro Salad with Arugula, Artichokes & Pistachios

Preparation Time: 15 minutes

Serves: 1

Calories: 350 **Carbs:** 45g **Protein:** 8g **Fat:** 15g **Fiber:** 8g
Sodium: 100mg

Ingredients:

1/2 cup farro, cooked

1 cup arugula

1/4 cup artichoke hearts, chopped

2 tablespoons pistachios, chopped

1 tablespoon olive oil

1 tablespoon lemon juice

1/2 teaspoon Dijon mustard

A pinch of salt

Method of Preparation:

1. In a bowl, combine farro, arugula, artichoke hearts, and pistachios.
2. In a small bowl, whisk together olive oil, lemon juice, Dijon mustard, salt.
3. Drizzle dressing over the salad and toss to combine.
4. Serve and enjoy!

Salmon-Stuffed Avocados

Preparation Time: 10 minutes

Serves: 1

Calories: 350 **Carbs:** 15g **Protein:** 30g **Fat:** 20g **Fiber:** 10g
Sodium: 100mg

Ingredients:

1 avocado, halved and pitted

4 oz cooked salmon, flaked

1/4 cup Greek yogurt

1/4 cup cucumber, diced

1/4 cup red onion, diced

1 tablespoon lemon juice

1 tablespoon dill, chopped

A pinch of salt

Method of Preparation:

1. In a bowl, combine salmon, Greek yogurt, cucumber,
    red onion, lemon juice, dill, and salt.

2. Spoon salmon mixture into avocado halves.

3. Serve and enjoy!

Winter Kale & Quinoa Salad with Avocado

Preparation Time: 15 minutes

Serves: 1

Calories: 400 **Carbs:** 40g **Protein:** 10g **Fat:** 25g **Fiber:** 10g **Sodium:** 100mg

Ingredients:

1 cup kale, chopped

1/2 cup cooked quinoa

1/4 cup pomegranate seeds

1/4 cup walnuts, chopped

1/4 avocado, diced

1 tablespoon olive oil

1 tablespoon balsamic vinegar

1/2 teaspoon honey

A pinch of salt

Method of Preparation:

1. In a bowl, combine kale, quinoa, pomegranate seeds, walnuts, and avocado.
2. In a small bowl, whisk together olive oil, balsamic vinegar, honey, salt.
3. Drizzle dressing over the salad and toss to combine.
4. Serve and enjoy!

Green Goddess Salad with Chickpeas

Preparation Time: 10 minutes

Serves: 1

Calories: 300 **Carbs:** 35g **Protein:** 10g **Fat:** 15g **Fiber:** 10g **Sodium:** 200mg

Ingredients:

2 cups mixed greens

1/2 cup chickpeas, drained and rinsed

1/4 cup cucumber, sliced

1/4 avocado, diced

2 tablespoons green goddess dressing

Method of Preparation:

1. In a large bowl, combine mixed greens, chickpeas, cucumber, and avocado.
2. Drizzle green goddess dressing over the salad and toss to combine.
3. Serve and enjoy!

DINNER

Chicken & Spinach Skillet Pasta with Lemon & Parmesan

Preparation Time: 30 minutes

Serves: 1

Calories: 450 **Carbs:** 45g **Protein:** 35g **Fat:** 15g **Fiber:** 5g **Sodium:** 90mg

Ingredients:

4 oz whole wheat pasta

4 oz chicken breast, diced

1 cup spinach

1/4 cup Parmesan cheese, grated

1 tablespoon olive oil

1 tablespoon lemon juice

1/2 teaspoon garlic powder

A pinch of salt

Method of Preparation:

1. Cook pasta according to package instructions, drain, and set aside.
2. In a skillet over medium heat, cook chicken in olive oil until browned and cooked through.
3. Add spinach, garlic powder, and salt to the skillet and cook until spinach is wilted.
4. Add cooked pasta, lemon juice, and Parmesan cheese to the skillet and toss to combine.
5. Serve hot.

Spinach & Mushroom Quiche

Preparation Time: 55 minutes

Serves: 6

Calories: 250 **Carbs:** 20g **Protein:** 10g **Fat:** 15g **Fiber:** 2g
Sodium: 100mg

Ingredients:

1 pre-made whole wheat pie crust

4 eggs

1 cup milk

1 cup spinach, chopped

1/2 cup mushrooms, sliced

1/4 cup red onion, diced

1/2 cup shredded cheddar cheese

1/2 teaspoon garlic powder

Method of Preparation:

1. Preheat oven to 350°F (175°C).

2. In a bowl, whisk together eggs, milk, and garlic powder.

3. Stir in spinach, mushrooms, red onion, and cheddar cheese.

4. Pour mixture into the pie crust and bake for 40-45 minutes, or until the quiche is set and the crust is golden brown.

5. Allow to cool slightly before slicing and serving.

Crispy Rice Bowls with Fried Eggs

Preparation Time: 20 minutes

Serves: 1

Calories: 400 **Carbs:** 40g **Protein:** 15g **Fat:** 20g **Fiber:** 10g **Sodium:** 100mg

Ingredients:

1 cup cooked brown rice

2 eggs

1/2 cup black beans, drained and rinsed

1/4 cup salsa

1/4 avocado, sliced

1 tablespoon olive oil

1/2 teaspoon garlic powder

A pinch of salt

Method of Preparation:

1. In a skillet over medium heat, heat olive oil.
2. Add cooked rice and spread it out in an even layer.
3. Cook without stirring for 5-7 minutes, or until the rice is crispy on the bottom.
4. In a separate skillet, fry eggs to desired doneness.
5. In a bowl, layer crispy rice, black beans, salsa, fried eggs, and avocado slices.
6. Serve hot.

Gochujang-Glazed Salmon with Garlic Spinach

Preparation Time: 30 minutes

Serves: 1

Calories: 350 **Carbs:** 15g **Protein:** 25g **Fat:** 20g **Fiber:** 2g **Sodium:** 50mg

Ingredients:

4 oz salmon fillet

1 tablespoon gochujang paste

1 tablespoon honey

1/2 tablespoon soy sauce

1 cup spinach

1 clove garlic, minced

1/2 tablespoon olive oil

A pinch of salt

Method of Preparation:

1. Preheat oven to 400°F (200°C).
2. In a small bowl, mix gochujang paste, honey, and soy sauce.
3. Place salmon fillet on a baking sheet lined with parchment paper and brush with the gochujang mixture.

4. Bake for 12-15 minutes, or until salmon is cooked through.

5. In a skillet, heat olive oil over medium heat.

6. Add garlic and sauté for 1-2 minutes.

7. Add spinach and cook until wilted.

8. Serve salmon over garlic spinach.

Broccoli & Quinoa Casserole

Preparation Time: 45 minutes

Serves: 4

Calories: 250 **Carbs:** 30g **Protein:** 12g **Fat:** 10g **Fiber:** 4g **Sodium:** 50mg

Ingredients:

1 cup cooked quinoa

1 cup broccoli florets, steamed

1/2 cup cheddar cheese, shredded

1/4 cup milk

1/4 cup Greek yogurt

1/4 cup breadcrumbs

1/2 teaspoon garlic powder

A pinch of salt

Method of Preparation:

1. Preheat oven to 375°F (190°C).
2. In a large bowl, mix cooked quinoa, steamed broccoli, cheddar cheese, milk, Greek yogurt, garlic powder, and salt.
3. Spread mixture in a baking dish and sprinkle breadcrumbs over the top.
4. Bake for 20-25 minutes, or until bubbly and golden brown.

Salmon with Lemon-Herb Orzo & Broccoli

Preparation Time: 30 minutes

Serves: 1

Calories: 400 **Carbs:** 30g **Protein:** 30g **Fat:** 18g **Fiber:** 4g
Sodium: 90mg

Ingredients:

4 oz salmon fillet

1/2 cup orzo, cooked

1 cup broccoli florets, steamed

1/2 tablespoon olive oil

1/2 tablespoon lemon juice

1/2 teaspoon dried basil

1/2 teaspoon dried oregano

A pinch of salt

Method of Preparation:

1. Season salmon fillet with olive oil, lemon juice, basil, oregano, and salt.
2. Grill or bake salmon until cooked through.
3. In a bowl, mix cooked orzo and steamed broccoli.
4. Serve salmon over lemon-herb orzo and broccoli mixture.

Easy Salmon Cakes with Arugula Salad

Preparation Time: 30 minutes

Serves: 2

Calories: 350 **Carbs:** 20g **Protein:** 30g **Fat:** 15g **Fiber:** 2g
Sodium: 600mg

Salmon Cakes:

1 can (14.75 oz) salmon, drained and flaked

1/2 cup breadcrumbs

1/4 cup Greek yogurt

1 egg

1 tablespoon Dijon mustard

1/2 teaspoon garlic powder

A pinch of salt

1 tablespoon olive oil

Arugula Salad:

2 cups arugula

1/4 cup cucumber, sliced

1/4 cup red onion, thinly sliced

1 tablespoon olive oil

1 tablespoon balsamic vinegar

A pinch of salt

Method of Preparation:

1. In a bowl, mix flaked salmon, breadcrumbs, Greek yogurt, egg, Dijon mustard, garlic powder, salt.
2. Form mixture into patties.
3. Heat olive oil in a skillet over medium heat.
4. Cook salmon cakes for 3-4 minutes per side, or until golden brown and cooked through.
5. In a bowl, combine arugula, cucumber, and red onion.
6. In a small bowl, whisk together olive oil, balsamic vinegar, salt.
7. Toss salad with dressing and serve with salmon cakes.

Salmon & Asparagus with Lemon-Garlic Butter Sauce

Preparation Time: 30 minutes

Serves: 1

Calories: 400 **Carbs:** 10g **Protein:** 25g **Fat:** 30g **Fiber:** 4g **Sodium:** 200mg

Ingredients:

4 oz salmon fillet

1/2 bunch asparagus, trimmed

1 tablespoon olive oil

1 tablespoon butter

1 clove garlic, minced

1 tablespoon lemon juice

1/2 teaspoon lemon zest

A pinch of salt

Method of Preparation:

1. Preheat oven to 400°F (200°C).

2. Place salmon fillet and asparagus on a baking sheet lined with parchment paper.

3. Drizzle with olive oil and season with salt.

4. Bake for 12-15 minutes, or until salmon is cooked through and asparagus is tender.

5. In a small saucepan, melt butter over medium heat.

6. Add garlic and cook for 1-2 minutes, or until fragrant.

7. Remove from heat and stir in lemon juice and zest.

8. Serve salmon and asparagus with lemon-garlic butter sauce.

Skillet Lemon Chicken with Spinach

Preparation Time: 30 minutes

Serves: 1

Calories: 300 **Carbs:** 5g **Protein:** 35g **Fat:** 15g **Fiber:** 2g **Sodium:** 100mg

Ingredients:

4 oz chicken breast

1/2 tablespoon olive oil

1 clove garlic, minced

1/2 lemon, juiced

1/2 teaspoon lemon zest

1/2 teaspoon dried oregano

A pinch of salt

2 cups spinach

Method of Preparation:

1. Season chicken breast with salt, and dried oregano.
2. Heat olive oil in a skillet over medium heat.
3. Add chicken breast and cook for 5-7 minutes per side, or until cooked through.
4. Remove chicken from skillet and set aside.
5. In the same skillet, add garlic and cook for 1-2 minutes, or until fragrant.
6. Add lemon juice and zest, scraping up any browned bits from the bottom of the skillet.
7. Add spinach to the skillet and cook until wilted.
8. Serve chicken over spinach.

Broccoli and Turkey Sausage Skillet Pizza

Preparation Time: 40 minutes

Serves: 4

Calories: 350 **Carbs:** 30g **Protein:** 20g **Fat:** 15g **Fiber:** 4g **Sodium:** 50mg

Ingredients:

1 pre-made whole wheat pizza crust

1 cup broccoli florets, steamed

1/2 cup turkey sausage, crumbled and cooked

1/2 cup shredded mozzarella cheese

1/2 teaspoon dried oregano

A pinch of salt

Method of Preparation:

1. Preheat oven to 425°F (220°C).
2. Place pizza crust on a baking sheet.

3. Top with broccoli, turkey sausage, and mozzarella cheese.

4. Sprinkle with dried oregano, salt, .

5. Bake for 12-15 minutes, or until cheese is melted and bubbly.

6. Slice and serve.

POULTRY MAINS

Lemon Chicken Skillet

Preparation Time: 40 minutes

Serves: 1

Calories: 250 **Carbs:** 2g **Protein:** 35g **Fat:** 10g **Fiber:** 1g **Sodium:** 100mg

Ingredients:

4 oz chicken breast

1/2 tablespoon olive oil

1 clove garlic, minced

1/2 lemon, juiced

1/2 teaspoon lemon zest

1/2 teaspoon dried thyme

A pinch of salt

Method of Preparation:

1. Season chicken breast with salt, and dried thyme.
2. Heat olive oil in a skillet over medium heat.
3. Add chicken breast and cook for 5-7 minutes per side, or until cooked through.
4. Remove chicken from skillet and set aside.
5. In the same skillet, add garlic and cook for 1-2 minutes, or until fragrant.
6. Add lemon juice and zest, scraping up any browned bits from the bottom of the skillet.
7. Return chicken to the skillet and coat with the lemon-garlic sauce.
8. Serve hot.

Chicken Enchilada Skillet Casserole

Preparation Time: 30 minutes

Serves: 2

Calories: 400 **Carbs:** 30g **Protein:** 25g **Fat:** 20g **Fiber:** 7g
Sodium: 60mg

Ingredients:

4 oz chicken breast, diced

1/4 cup onion, diced

1/2 cup black beans, drained and rinsed

1/2 cup corn kernels

1/2 cup enchilada sauce

1/2 cup shredded cheddar cheese

1/2 teaspoon chili powder

1/2 teaspoon cumin

A pinch of salt

1 tablespoon olive oil

Method of Preparation:

1. Heat olive oil in a skillet over medium heat.
2. Add chicken breast and cook until browned.
3. Add onion and cook until its softened.
4. Stir in black beans, corn, enchilada sauce, chili powder, cumin, salt.
5. Sprinkle shredded cheddar cheese over the top.

6. Cover and cook for 5-7 minutes, or until cheese is melted and bubbly.

7. Serve hot.

Chicken Paprikash with Mushrooms & Onions

Preparation Time: 30 minutes

Serves: 1

Calories: 300 **Carbs:** 10g **Protein:** 35g **Fat:** 15g **Fiber:** 3g **Sodium:** 90mg

Ingredients:

4 oz chicken breast

1/2 onion, sliced

1/2 cup mushrooms, sliced

1/2 cup chicken broth

1/4 cup Greek yogurt

1 tablespoon paprika

1/2 teaspoon garlic powder

A pinch of salt

1 tablespoon olive oil

Method of Preparation:

1. Season chicken breast with paprika, garlic powder, salt, .
2. Heat olive oil in a skillet over medium heat.
3. Add chicken breast and cook for 5-7 minutes per side, or until cooked through.
4. Remove chicken from skillet and set aside.
5. In the same skillet, add onion and mushrooms, and cook until softened.
6. Stir in chicken broth and Greek yogurt, and bring to a simmer.
7. Return chicken to the skillet and coat with the sauce.
8. Serve hot.

Chicken with Farro

Preparation Time: 30 minutes

Serves: 1

Calories: 400 **Carbs:** 45g **Protein:** 35g **Fat:** 10g **Fiber:** 8g
Sodium: 100mg

Ingredients:

4 oz chicken breast

1/2 cup farro, cooked

1/2 cup broccoli florets, steamed

1/4 cup onion, diced

1 clove garlic, minced

1/2 tablespoon olive oil

1/2 lemon, juiced

1/2 teaspoon dried oregano

A pinch of salt

Method of Preparation:

1. Season chicken breast with salt, and dried oregano.
2. Heat olive oil in a skillet over medium heat.
3. Add chicken breast and cook for 5-7 minutes per side, or until cooked through.
4. Remove chicken from skillet and set aside.
5. In the same skillet, add onion and garlic, and cook until softened.

6. Add cooked farro, broccoli, and lemon juice to the skillet.

7. Cook for another 2-3 minutes, or until heated through.

8. Serve chicken over farro mixture.

Chicken Cutlets with Brussels Sprouts

Preparation Time: 35 minutes

Serves: 1

Calories: 400 **Carbs:** 30g **Protein:** 35g **Fat:** 15g **Fiber:** 5g **Sodium:** 400mg

Ingredients:

4 oz chicken breast, pounded thin

1/2 cup breadcrumbs

1/4 cup Parmesan cheese, grated

1 egg, beaten

1/2 cup Brussels sprouts, halved

1/4 cup red onion, sliced

1 clove garlic, minced

1/2 tablespoon olive oil

1/2 lemon, juiced

A pinch of salt

Method of Preparation:

1. In a bowl, mix breadcrumbs and Parmesan cheese.
2. Dip chicken breast in beaten egg, then coat with breadcrumb mixture.
3. Heat olive oil in a skillet over medium heat.
4. Add chicken breast and cook for 3-4 minutes per side, or until golden brown and cooked through.
5. Remove chicken from skillet and set aside.
6. In the same skillet, add Brussels sprouts, red onion, and garlic, and cook until vegetables are tender.
7. Stir in lemon juice, and salt.
8. Serve chicken cutlets with Brussels sprouts mixture.

SEAFOOD MAINS

Seafood Roast with Smoky Garlic Butter

Preparation Time: 30 minutes

Serves: 1

Calories: 400 **Carbs:** 10g **Protein:** 35g **Fat:** 25g **Fiber:** 2g **Sodium:** 100mg

Ingredients:

4 oz shrimp, peeled and deveined

4 oz scallops

4 oz salmon fillet

1/2 tablespoon olive oil

1/2 tablespoon smoked paprika

1/2 tablespoon garlic powder

A pinch of salt

1/2 lemon, juiced

1/2 teaspoon lemon zest

1 clove garlic, minced

1 tablespoon butter

Method of Preparation:

1. Preheat oven to 400°F (200°C).
2. Place shrimp, scallops, and salmon fillet on a baking sheet lined with parchment paper.
3. Drizzle with olive oil and sprinkle with smoked paprika, garlic powder, and salt.
4. Bake for 10-12 minutes, or until seafood is cooked through.
5. In a small saucepan, melt butter over medium heat.
6. Add lemon juice, lemon zest, and minced garlic.
7. Cook for 1-2 minutes, or until garlic is fragrant.
8. Drizzle garlic butter over roasted seafood.

Crab and Asparagus Pappardelle

Preparation Time: 30 minutes

Serves: 1

Calories: 400 **Carbs:** 45g **Protein:** 25g **Fat:** 15g **Fiber:** 5g
Sodium: 300mg

Ingredients:

4 oz pappardelle pasta, cooked

4 oz crab meat

1/2 cup asparagus, chopped

1/4 cup onion, diced

1 clove garlic, minced

1/2 tablespoon olive oil

1/2 lemon, juiced

A pinch of salt

1 tablespoon Parmesan cheese, grated

Method of Preparation:

1. In a skillet, heat olive oil over medium heat.
2. Add asparagus, onion, and garlic.
3. Cook for 5-7 minutes, or until vegetables are tender.
4. Add crab meat and cook for another 2-3 minutes, or until heated through.

5. Stir in cooked pappardelle pasta and lemon juice.

6. Season with salt.

7. Serve hot, sprinkled with Parmesan cheese.

Cheesy Seafood Bake

Preparation Time: 30 minutes

Serves: 2

Calories: 400 **Carbs:** 15g **Protein:** 35g **Fat:** 20g **Fiber:** 3g **Sodium:** 100mg

Ingredients:

4 oz white fish fillet

4 oz shrimp, peeled and deveined

4 oz crab meat

1/4 cup red onion, sliced

1/4 cup black olives, sliced

1/2 cup marinara sauce

1/2 cup shredded mozzarella cheese

1/2 teaspoon dried oregano

A pinch of salt

Method of Preparation:

1. Preheat oven to 375°F (190°C).
2. Place white fish fillet, shrimp, and crab meat in a baking dish.
3. Top with red onion, and black olives.
4. Pour marinara sauce over the seafood and vegetables.
5. Sprinkle with shredded mozzarella cheese and dried oregano.
6. Bake for 15-20 minutes, or until cheese is melted and bubbly.
7. Serve hot.

Lobster with Thermidor Butter

Preparation Time: 30 minutes

Serves: 1

Calories: 300 **Carbs:** 2g **Protein:** 25g **Fat:** 20g **Fiber:** 0g

Sodium: 400mg

Ingredients:

1 lobster tail

1/2 tablespoon olive oil

1/2 tablespoon butter

1 clove garlic, minced

1/2 tablespoon Dijon mustard

1/4 cup heavy cream

1/4 cup Parmesan cheese, grated

1/2 teaspoon paprika

A pinch of salt

1/2 lemon, juiced

Method of Preparation:

1. Preheat oven to 375°F (190°C).
2. Using kitchen shears, cut the top of the lobster shell to expose the meat.
3. Drizzle lobster tail with olive oil and season with salt.
4. Roast lobster tail for 12-15 minutes, or until meat is opaque and cooked through.
5. In a saucepan, melt butter over medium heat.
6. Add minced garlic and cook for 1-2 minutes, or until fragrant.

7. Stir in Dijon mustard, heavy cream, Parmesan cheese, paprika, and salt.

8. Cook for another 2-3 minutes, or until sauce is thickened.

9. Stir in lemon juice.

10. Serve lobster tail with Thermidor butter sauce.

Roasted Salmon with Asparagus

Preparation Time: 30 minutes

Serves: 1

Calories: 350 **Carbs:** 10g **Protein:** 25g **Fat:** 20g **Fiber:** 5g **Sodium:** 100mg

Ingredients:

4 oz salmon fillet

1/2 bunch asparagus, trimmed

1/2 tablespoon olive oil

1/2 lemon, juiced

1/2 teaspoon lemon zest

1/2 teaspoon dried dill

A pinch of salt

Method of Preparation:

1. Preheat oven to 400°F (200°C).
2. Place salmon fillet and asparagus on a baking sheet lined with parchment paper.
3. Drizzle with olive oil and season with salt, dried dill, lemon juice, and lemon zest.
4. Bake for 12-15 minutes, or until salmon is cooked through and asparagus is tender.
5. Serve hot.

SMOOTHIES

Raspberry-Peach-Mango Smoothie Bowl

Preparation Time: 5 minutes

Serves: 1

Calories: 250 **Carbs:** 45g **Protein:** 10g **Fat:** 4g **Fiber:** 8g
Sodium: 50mg

Ingredients:

1/2 cup frozen raspberries

1/2 cup frozen peach slices

1/2 cup frozen mango chunks

1/2 cup Greek yogurt

1/4 cup almond milk

1 tablespoon honey

Toppings: fresh raspberries, sliced peaches, sliced mangoes, granola, chia seeds

Method of Preparation:

1. In a blender, combine frozen raspberries, peach slices, mango chunks, Greek yogurt, almond milk, and honey.
2. Blend until smooth.
3. Pour into a bowl and top with fresh raspberries, sliced peaches, sliced mangoes, granola, and chia seeds.

Peanut Butter & Jelly Smoothie

Preparation Time: 5 minutes

Serves: 1

Calories: 300 **Carbs:** 40g **Protein:** 7g **Fat:** 14g **Fiber:** 6g
Sodium: 100mg

Ingredients:

1/2 cup frozen mixed berries

1/2 banana

1 tablespoon peanut butter

1/2 cup almond milk

1 tablespoon honey

Method of Preparation:

1. In a blender, combine frozen mixed berries, banana, peanut butter, almond milk, and honey.
2. Blend until smooth.

Mango-Almond Smoothie Bowl

Preparation Time: 5 minutes

Serves: 1

Calories: 250 **Carbs:** 30g **Protein:** 5g **Fat:** 14g **Fiber:** 5g **Sodium:** 50mg

Ingredients:

1/2 cup frozen mango chunks

1/2 banana

1/2 cup almond milk

1 tablespoon almond butter

Toppings: sliced almonds, fresh mango chunks, granola, chia seeds

Method of Preparation:

1. In a blender, combine frozen mango chunks, banana, almond milk, and almond butter.
2. Blend until smooth.
3. Pour into a bowl and top with sliced almonds, fresh mango chunks, granola, and chia seeds.

Strawberry-Banana Green Smoothie

Preparation Time: 5 minutes

Serves: 1

Calories: 150 **Carbs:** 35g **Protein:** 3g **Fat:** 2g **Fiber:** 5g **Sodium:** 100mg

Ingredients:

1/2 cup strawberries, hulled

1/2 banana

1 cup spinach

1/2 cup almond milk

1 tablespoon honey

Method of Preparation:

1. In a blender, combine strawberries, banana, spinach, almond milk, and honey.
2. Blend until smooth.

Blackberry Smoothie

Preparation Time: 5 minutes

Serves: 1

Calories: 200 **Carbs:** 40g **Protein:** 10g **Fat:** 2g **Fiber:** 8g **Sodium:** 100mg

Ingredients:

1/2 cup blackberries

1/2 banana

1/2 cup Greek yogurt

1/2 cup almond milk

1 tablespoon honey

Method of Preparation:

1. In a blender, combine blackberries, banana, Greek yogurt, almond milk, and honey.

2. Blend until smooth.

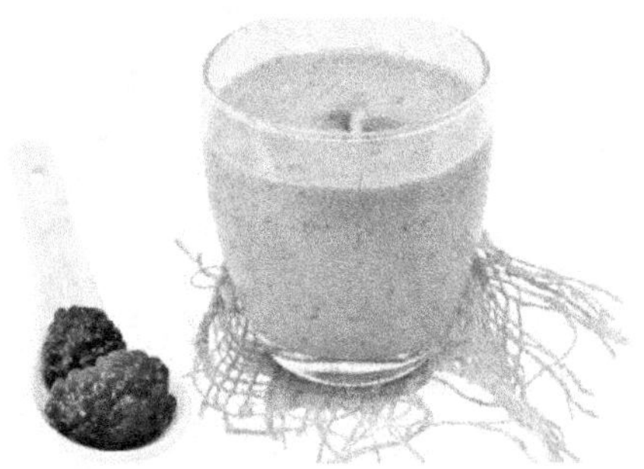

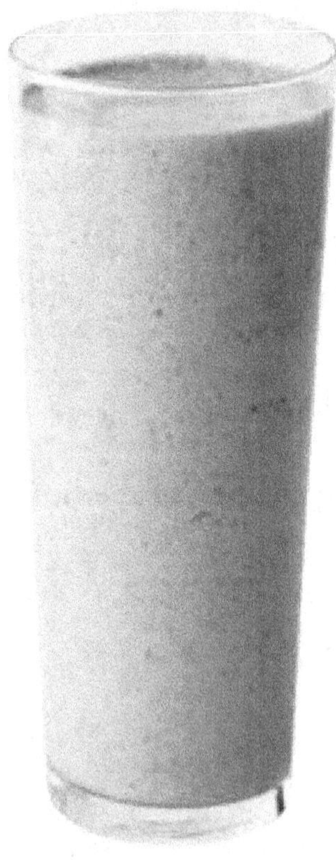

CONCLUSION

In conclusion, a Rheumatoid Arthritis diet plays a crucial role in managing the symptoms and progression of the disease.

By focusing on anti-inflammatory foods and avoiding those that can exacerbate inflammation, you can potentially reduce pain, stiffness, and joint damage associated with Rheumatoid Arthritis.

The diet emphasizes whole, nutrient-dense foods such as fruits, vegetables, whole grains, lean proteins, and healthy fats.

These foods are rich in antioxidants and other compounds that help reduce inflammation in the body.

Additionally, incorporating anti-inflammatory herbs and spices like turmeric, ginger, and cinnamon can provide added benefits.

On the other hand, foods high in sugar, refined carbohydrates, and saturated fats should be limited, as they can promote inflammation. Reducing the intake of processed foods, fried foods, and sugary beverages is also recommended.

Following an anti-inflammatory diet can offer numerous benefits for seniors with Rheumatoid Arthritis.

It can help improve joint function, reduce pain and swelling, and enhance overall quality of life. Additionally, maintaining a healthy weight through diet can alleviate pressure on the joints, further reducing symptoms.

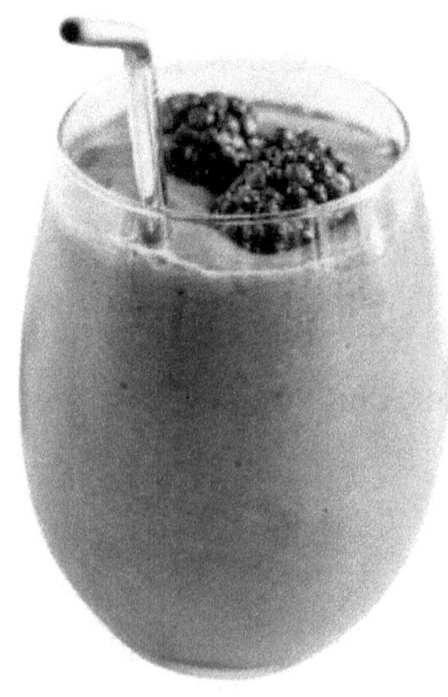

www.ingramcontent.com/pod-product-compliance
Lightning Source LLC
Chambersburg PA
CBHW050825250726
48653CB00006B/2427